DETOX IN THREE

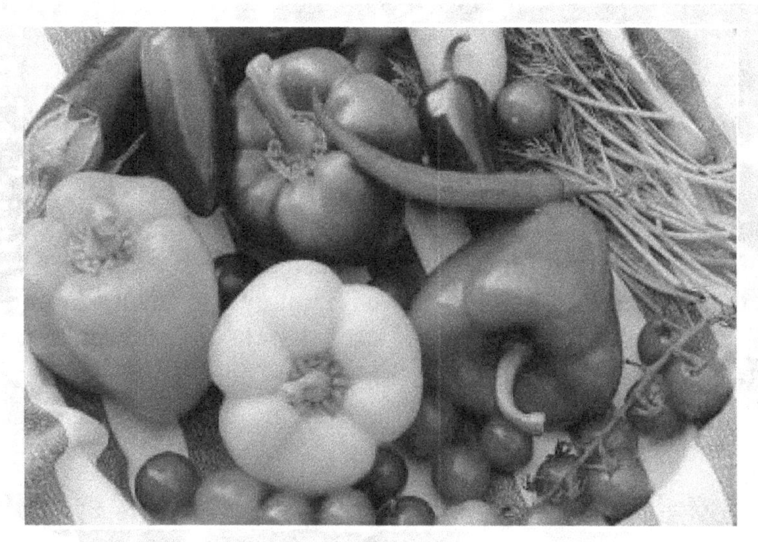

The Ultimate Guide to Body Renewal

D.C Kelly

TABLE OF CONTENTS

INTRODUCTION

Welcome to "Detox in Three!" your profound journey to a rejuvenated and revitalized version of you! We will go on an extraordinary three-day detox trip with this detailed guide. Prepare to be transformed to maximum health, increased energy, and a revitalized sense of self.

Are you searching for a way to give your body and mind a reset? Do you long for an in-depth plan for wellness that is fun, attainable, and effective? There's nowhere else to look! This book is your stepping stone to a rejuvenating experience that will give you motivation, resilience, and the confidence to begin your journey to a more vibrant lifestyle.

Imagine an adventure where you get closer to a lighter body, a brighter mind, and a dazzling radiance every day. "Detox in Three" is a life-changing book that aims to awaken your senses and fuel your desire for a better, happier version of yourself. It's not just a detox guide.

Within these pages, you will learn:

Delectable Detox dishes: Savour delectable dishes high in nutrients and designed to detoxify your body while stimulating your taste buds.

Empowering Daily Practices: Every day offers the opportunity to develop constructive habits that will remain effective long after your three-day trip, from morning routines to night-time reflections.

Professional Advice: The material in this program is carefully chosen and supported by the most recent wellness discoveries, guaranteeing that you receive expert guidance on movement, mindfulness, and nutrition.

Personalized Approach: Tailor the program to your unique preferences and lifestyle, making your detox experience not just effective but enjoyable.

Prepare yourself for an exciting journey towards a healthier, vibrant version of yourself. "Revitalize in Three" is more than simply a book- it is your travel companion as you find the potential that both your body and mind possess.

Are you ready to revitalize your body in three days? Let the adventure begin!

CHAPTER ONE

The Fundamentals of Detox

What is Detox?

Detoxification, or detox, is the process through which the body gets rid of or neutralizes dangerous compounds known as toxins. Toxins can originate from external sources such as diet, lifestyle, and environment. They can also be internal by-products of metabolism. The main objective of detoxification is to strengthen the body's inherent processes in getting rid of these potentially dangerous toxins.

Dietary adjustments, lifestyle adjustments, and exercises that help the organs involved in detoxification—are components of detox programs. Although the body contains natural detoxing mechanisms, there are extra measures that can enhance these functions and enhance general health.

The Effects of Toxins on the Body

Toxins can affect the body in several ways, sometimes resulting in health problems. Toxin effects are contingent upon various elements, including the kind of toxin, its concentration, and the individual's vulnerability. The following are a few common impacts of toxins:

Cell Damage: Certain toxins can harm cell structures, preventing regular cellular activity and possibly resulting in chronic illnesses.

Inflammatory Response: Toxins have the potential to cause an inflammatory response in the body, which can aggravate autoimmune disorders, cardiovascular diseases, and arthritis.

Reduced Metabolism: Some toxins can disrupt metabolic functions, impacting the synthesis of energy, the absorption of nutrients, and the overall balance of metabolism.

Organ Dysfunction: Extended exposure to toxins can cause the liver and kidneys, two organs involved in detoxification, to malfunction, making it more difficult for them to get rid of waste.

Reduced Immune Response: The immune system may be weakened by toxins, leaving the body more vulnerable to diseases and infections.

The Functions of Organs in Detox

Numerous organs are essential to the body's inherent detoxifying activities. Together, these organs help the body recognize, neutralize, and get rid of toxins:

Liver: The liver serves as the main organ for detoxification. Toxins are broken down into substances soluble in water and discharged through bile or urine.

Kidneys: Urine is a waste product and poison that the kidneys remove from the body after filtering the blood. They are essential for preserving electrolyte equilibrium.

Lungs: Through respiration, the lungs get rid of volatile poisons. Certain waste materials get expelled from the body through breathing out.

Skin: Sweating is how the body's largest organ, the skin, eliminates pollutants. Exercise and saunas can help the skin eliminate toxins.

Knowing how the body naturally detoxifies emphasizes how crucial it is to maintain these organs with a healthy, balanced lifestyle. Detox programs can help to achieve short-term objectives, but sustaining total well-being requires forming long-term behaviors that support the well-being of these vital organs. Remember to always consult a medical professional before beginning a detox program.

CHAPTER TWO

Benefits of Detoxing Your Body

1. Improved Digestive Health and Digestion

Improved Nutrient Absorption: Eating foods high in nutrients, which promote optimal nutrient absorption in the digestive tract, is a recommendation of detox programs.

Balanced microbiota: Detox can support a healthy, balanced gut microbiota vital for digestion, by encouraging the consumption of probiotics and foods high in fiber.

2. Increased Vitality and Energy

Toxin Elimination: The goal of detoxification is to get rid of substances that could be causing you to feel worn out and sluggish, which could give you more energy.

Nutritious Foods: Consuming foods high in nutrients, which boost general vitality and offer sustained energy, is a common focus of detox diets.

3. Focus and Mental Clarity

Detox programs can help reduce brain fog by removing foods and substances that can cause it, leading to an improvement in mental clarity.

Incorporation of Brain-Boosting Nutrients: Including foods rich in omega-3 fatty acids, antioxidants, and vitamins can support brain health and focus.

4. *Weight Management and Metabolism Boost*

Elimination of Processed Foods: Detox often involves reducing or eliminating processed and sugary foods, which can contribute to weight management.

Balanced Blood Sugar: Detox diets may help regulate blood sugar levels, supporting a balanced metabolism and weight management.

5. *Radiant Skin and Overall Well-being*

Hydration: Detox programs typically emphasize increased water intake, contributing to skin hydration and a healthy complexion.

Antioxidant-Rich Foods: Detox diets rich in antioxidants can combat oxidative stress, promoting skin health and overall well-being.

CHAPTER THREE

Effects of Detox

Short-Term Effects

1. Initial Fatigue: People may feel a decrease in energy or initial fatigue as their bodies adjust to dietary and lifestyle changes.

Management: To reduce fatigue, make sure you drink enough water, give rest priority, and make small adjustments over time.

2. Digestive Modifications: Temporary digestive modifications, such as bloating or increased bowel movements, can be brought on by dietary pattern alterations, increased fibre consumption, or the removal of foods.

Management: Drink plenty of water, eat foods high in fibre gradually, and be aware of your tolerance.

3. Mood Swings: Hormone imbalances brought on by detoxification procedures may cause irritability or mood swings.

Management: Take part in mindfulness exercises, stress-relieving activities, and share any emotional shifts with a support network.

4. Headaches: Detox programmes can cause headaches by dehydrating the body, changing blood sugar levels, or causing coffee withdrawal.

Management: Stay well-hydrated, gradually reduce caffeine intake, and maintain balanced blood sugar levels.

5. Temporary Weight Loss: Initial weight loss may occur due to water weight reduction, decreased inflammation, and changes in dietary patterns.

Management: Monitor weight changes, focus on long-term goals, and ensure nutritional needs are met.

Long-Term Effects

1. Improved Metabolism: Establishing healthier eating habits and regular physical activity can contribute to a sustained boost in metabolism over the long term.

Management: Maintain a balanced diet, engage in regular exercise, and prioritize overall well-being.

2. Sustained Energy Levels: Long-term adherence to a healthful lifestyle can lead to sustained energy levels as the body adapts to nutrient-rich foods and consistent physical activity.

Management: Continue to prioritize balanced nutrition, stay hydrated, and engage in regular exercise.

3. Weight Maintenance: Establishing healthy habits and balanced eating patterns can contribute to long-term weight maintenance.

Management: Focus on sustainable dietary choices, portion control, and regular physical activity.

Sustainable well-being is achieved through a balanced and holistic approach, encompassing nutrition, physical activity, stress management, and adequate sleep. Responses to detox can vary, and long-term effects depend on individual factors, adherence to healthy habits, and overall lifestyle.

CHAPTER FOUR

Taking Caution

While detox programs can offer benefits for many individuals, there are situations where detox may not be suitable or should be approached with caution. It's important to consider individual health conditions, medical history, and specific circumstances. Here are some situations where detox may not be advisable or should be discussed with a healthcare professional:

When Detox May Not Be Suitable

1. Pregnancy and Breastfeeding

Caution: Detox programs that involve significant dietary changes or restrictions may not be suitable for pregnant or breastfeeding individuals.

Consideration: Consult with a healthcare professional to determine safe practices that support both maternal and fatal health.

2. Underlying Health Conditions:

Caution: Individuals with certain health conditions such as eating disorders, kidney diseases, or liver disorders may need to exercise caution with detox programs.

Consideration: Prioritize personalized approaches and consult with a healthcare professional to ensure the detox plan aligns with individual health needs.

3. Medical Treatments

Caution: Individuals undergoing medical treatments or taking medications may need to avoid detox programs that could interfere with treatment efficacy.

Consideration: Coordinate with healthcare providers to integrate detox practices safely into the overall treatment plan.

4. Children and Adolescents

Caution: Detox programs that involve restrictive diets may not be suitable for children and adolescents, as they have specific nutritional requirements for growth and development.

Consideration: Focus on promoting a balanced and nutrient-rich diet suitable for their age and developmental stage.

Pre-existing Health Conditions and Detox

1. Liver or Kidney Disorders

Caution: Individuals with liver or kidney disorders should approach detox programs with caution, as these organs play a crucial role in detoxification.

Consideration: Consult with healthcare professionals to tailor detox plans that support organ function without causing harm.

2. Digestive Disorders

Caution: Those with digestive disorders, such as irritable bowel syndrome (IBS) or inflammatory bowel diseases, may need to be cautious with certain detox practices.

Consideration: Choose gentle detox methods and work with healthcare professionals to address specific dietary needs.

3. Heart Conditions

Caution: Detox programs that involve extreme dietary changes or fasting may pose risks for individuals with heart conditions or cardiovascular issues.

Consideration: Consult with cardiologists or healthcare professionals to develop a safe and suitable approach.

4. Diabetes

Caution: Detox programs that impact blood sugar levels may require careful consideration for individuals with diabetes.

Consideration: Work with healthcare professionals to modify detox plans to align with blood sugar management strategies.

Consulting with a Healthcare Professional

Individual Health Assessment

Caution: Before starting any detox program, it's essential to undergo an individual health assessment with a healthcare professional.

Consideration: Discuss pre-existing health conditions, medical history, and individual health goals to determine the suitability of a detox plan.

Monitoring Vital Signs

Caution: Regular monitoring of vital signs, blood parameters, and organ function is crucial during detox, especially for individuals with pre-existing health conditions.

Consideration: Establish a monitoring plan with healthcare professionals to ensure safety throughout the detox process.

Remember that individual health needs vary, and a one-size-fits-all approach may not be suitable. Consulting with healthcare professionals is essential to tailor detox plans that align with individual health goals while prioritizing safety and well-being.

CHAPTER FIVE

Planning Your Three-Day Detox Program

Setting Clear Goals

Define Your Objectives

Importance: Clearly articulate the specific goals you aim to achieve through the detox program.

Steps: Identify whether your goals focus on weight management, improved energy, mental clarity, or other health aspects. Establish measurable and realistic targets to track progress.

Prioritize Health and Well-being

Importance: Ensure that your goals prioritize overall health and well-being rather than solely focusing on rapid weight loss or short-term outcomes.

Steps: Emphasize goals related to enhanced energy, improved digestion, and mental clarity.

Consider Long-Term Impact

Importance: Frame goals in a way that promotes long-term lifestyle changes rather than temporary solutions.

Steps: Reflect on how the detox program can contribute to sustained well-being beyond the immediate timeframe.

Personalize Your Goals

Importance: Tailor goals to your individual needs, considering your current health status, preferences, and motivations.

Steps: Consider factors such as dietary preferences, activity levels, and any specific health concerns.

Preparing Your Body for Detox

Gradual Transition

Importance: Ease into the detox process by gradually reducing processed foods, caffeine, and other potential triggers.

Steps: Start incorporating more whole foods into your diet before the official detox period begins.

Stay Hydrated

Importance: Hydration is crucial for supporting the body's natural detoxification processes.

Steps: Increase water intake in the days leading up to the detox program.

Nutrient-Rich Foods

Importance: Ensure your body receives essential nutrients by focusing on a balanced diet rich in fruits, vegetables, lean proteins, and whole grains.

Steps: Include a variety of nutrient-dense foods to prepare your body for the upcoming dietary changes.

Limit Stimulants and Processed Foods

Importance: Gradually reduce the consumption of stimulants like caffeine and processed foods to minimize potential withdrawal symptoms.

Steps: Replace caffeinated beverages with herbal teas and minimize intake of processed and sugary foods.

Creating a Supportive Environment

Inform Your Support System

Importance: Share your detox goals with friends, family, or a support network to create accountability and understanding.

Steps: Communicate your intentions, potential challenges, and how they can offer support.

Clear Your Environment

Importance: Remove temptations and unhealthy foods from your home to create an environment that aligns with your detox goals.

Steps: Clean out your pantry and refrigerator, discarding or donating items that don't align with your plan.

Plan Meals and Snacks

Importance: Plan and prepare detox-friendly meals and snacks to make healthy choices easily accessible.

Steps: Create a meal plan for the detox period, incorporating a variety of nutrient-rich foods.

Establish Routine and Rituals

Importance: Incorporate daily routines and rituals that support your well-being, such as regular mealtimes, exercise sessions, and relaxation practices.

Steps: Create a daily schedule that includes time for nourishing activities and self-care.

By setting clear goals, preparing your body gradually and creating a supportive environment, you lay the foundation for a successful and sustainable detox journey. Remember that individual needs and preferences vary, so adapt these steps to align with your unique circumstances and consult with healthcare professionals for personalized guidance.

CHAPTER SIX

Your Three-Day Detox Menu

Day 1: Cleansing Start

Morning

Begin the day with a glass of warm water and lemon to kickstart digestion.

Breakfast: Include a green smoothie with spinach, kale, cucumber, and a touch of ginger.

Mid-Morning Snack: Eat a handful of raw almonds or walnuts for a nutrient boost.

Afternoon

Lunch: Have a colorful salad with mixed greens, tomatoes, avocado, and a light olive oil and lemon dressing.

Snack: Enjoy a refreshing cucumber and mint detox water.

Evening

Evening: Opt for a warm bowl of vegetable soup with nutrient-dense ingredients like broccoli, carrots, and kale.

Dinner: Choose a light and steamed protein source such as grilled chicken or fish, paired with steamed vegetables.

Before Bed: Sip on a cup of chamomile tea to promote relaxation.

Day 2: Nutrient Boost

Morning

Begin with a green tea rich in antioxidants.

Breakfast: Prepare a nutrient-packed smoothie with berries, banana, chia seeds, and a scoop of plant-based protein powder.

Mid-Morning Snack: Snack on a piece of fresh fruit like an apple or pear.

Afternoon

Lunch: Enjoy a quinoa or brown rice bowl with mixed vegetables and a tahini dressing.

Snack: Have a handful of pumpkin seeds for added nutrients.

Evening

Evening: Prepare a light and colorful stir-fry with a variety of veggies and tofu.

Dinner: Opt for a grilled salmon fillet with a side of steamed broccoli and quinoa.

Before Bed: Try a cup of peppermint tea to aid digestion.

Day 3: Renew and Recharge

Start with a detoxifying herbal tea like dandelion or ginger.

Breakfast: Make a smoothie with pineapple, kiwi, and mint for a refreshing start.

Mid-Morning Snack: Snack on a small bowl of mixed berries.

Afternoon

Lunch: Create a vibrant salad with mixed greens, watermelon, feta cheese, and a balsamic vinaigrette.

Snack: Have a piece of dark chocolate for a touch of antioxidants.

Evening

Evening: Prepare a light vegetable and lentil soup for dinner.

Dinner: Opt for a grilled portobello mushroom cap stuffed with quinoa and roasted vegetables.

Before Bed: Enjoy a cup of herbal chamomile or lavender tea to promote relaxation.

Remember to stay hydrated throughout each day by drinking plenty of water, herbal teas, and detox waters. Additionally, listen to your body's cues and make necessary adjustments.

CHAPTER SEVEN

Detox Program Guidelines

Hydration, detox-friendly foods and herbal teas play integral roles in supporting the body's natural detoxification processes.

Hydration and Detox

Water

Importance: Proper hydration is essential for overall health and supports the body's detoxification processes by aiding in the elimination of toxins.

Recommendation: Drink at least 8 glasses (64 ounces) of water per day, and more if engaging in physical activity.

Detox Waters

Ingredients:

Cucumber slices
Lemon or lime wedges
Fresh mint leaves

How to Prepare: Combine the ingredients in a pitcher of water and let it infuse overnight for a refreshing detox water.

Importance: Coconut water is not only hydrating but also rich in electrolytes, supporting overall hydration.

Recommendation: Include coconut water as a hydrating beverage during the day.

Detox-Friendly Foods

Leafy Greens

Examples: Spinach, kale, Swiss chard

Benefits: Rich in chlorophyll, these greens support liver function, which is crucial for detoxification.

Cruciferous Vegetables

Examples: Broccoli, cauliflower, Brussels sprouts

Benefits: High in antioxidants and sulfur-containing compounds, aiding the liver in detox processes.

Berries

Examples: Blueberries, strawberries, raspberries

Benefits: Packed with antioxidants that combat oxidative stress and inflammation.

Citrus Fruits

Examples: Oranges, lemons, grapefruits

Benefits: High in vitamin C, supporting the production of glutathione, an antioxidant crucial for detoxification.

Turmeric

Benefits: Contains curcumin, which has anti-inflammatory and antioxidant properties, supporting overall detox.

Garlic

Benefits: Contains sulfur compounds that assist the liver in detoxification processes.

Avocado

Benefits: Provides healthy fats and supports the body's production of glutathione.

Herbal Teas and Infusions

Dandelion Tea

Benefits: Acts as a natural diuretic, promoting kidney function and supporting detoxification.

Ginger Tea

Benefits: Has anti-inflammatory properties and aids digestion, supporting the gastrointestinal tract during detox.

Peppermint Tea

Benefits: Relaxes the digestive tract and helps alleviate bloating and gas.

Green Tea

Benefits: Rich in antioxidants, particularly catechins, which support cellular health.

Chamomile Tea

Benefits: Known for its calming effects, chamomile tea can help reduce stress and promote better sleep.

Nettle Tea

Benefits: Supports kidney function and provides essential nutrients like vitamins and minerals.

Lemon Balm Infusion

Benefits: Calming and soothing, lemon balm can contribute to stress reduction during detox.

Remember to incorporate a variety of these foods and beverages into your daily routine to support a well-rounded detox.

CHAPTER EIGHT

Tracking Your Progress

Journaling

Daily Entries

Record your daily experiences, including meals, snacks, and beverages consumed. Note any physical symptoms or changes you observe, such as energy levels, digestion, and sleep quality.

Food Diary

Document the detox-friendly foods you include in your meals. Track portion sizes and note how your body responds to different foods.

Emotional Well-Being

Express your emotions and feelings throughout the detox process. Note any emotional triggers or patterns related to food or lifestyle choices.

Goals and Intentions

Write down your detox goals and intentions at the beginning of each day. Reflect on how much progress you have made and celebrate the little wins.

Gratitude Journal

Include a section for gratitude, noting positive aspects of your detox experience. Acknowledge your progress and be grateful for the support you receive.

Reflection

Physical Changes

Regularly assess and reflect on any physical changes you observe. Note improvements in energy levels, skin complexion, or changes in weight.

Digestive Health

Reflect on changes in digestion, including any improvements or challenges. Note how certain foods impact your digestive well-being.

Mood and Mental Clarity

Evaluate changes in mood, stress levels, and mental clarity. Identify factors contributing to mental well-being or areas that need attention.

Sleep Patterns

Reflect on sleep quality and any changes in your sleep patterns. Note factors influencing your ability to rest well.

Cravings and Habits

Identify any cravings or habits that arise during the detox. Reflect on strategies to manage cravings and make healthier choices.

Challenges and Solutions

Document challenges encountered during the detox. Reflect on effective solutions and adjustments to overcome obstacles.

Self-Discovery

Use journaling as a tool for self-discovery. Reflect on your relationship with food, stressors, and how your body responds to different stimuli.

Mindful Eating Reflection

Practice mindful eating and reflect on the experience. Note sensations, flavors, and the impact on overall satisfaction.

Tips for Effective Journaling and Reflection

Be Honest and Authentic

Write openly about how you have felt and what you have experienced.

Set Regular Times

Establish a routine for journaling, whether it's in the morning, evening, or both.

Use Prompts

Utilize prompts to guide your reflections and ensure a comprehensive assessment.

Track Progress

Review previous entries to track progress and identify patterns.

Celebrate Achievements

Celebrate your wins, regardless of how small they may be.

Adapt as Needed

Adjust your journaling approach based on your evolving needs and experiences.

By incorporating journaling and reflection into your detox journey, you'll gain valuable insights, foster self-awareness, and stay connected to your goals. It can serve as a source of motivation, helping you make informed decisions about your health and well-being.

CHAPTER NINE

Post-Detox Transition

Gradually reintroducing foods after a detox and maintaining its benefits in daily life are crucial steps to ensure a sustainable and healthy transition. Here's a guide on how to approach the reintroduction of foods and sustain the positive effects of detox in your daily routine:

Gradual Reintroduction of Foods

Start with Whole Foods

Begin by reintroducing whole, minimally processed foods. Focus on nutrient-dense options such as fruits, vegetables, lean proteins, and whole grains.

One at a Time

Introduce one food group at a time to monitor how your body reacts. This helps identify any specific sensitivities or reactions.

Observe Reactions

Pay attention to how your body responds to each reintroduced food. Look for changes in energy levels, digestion, skin health, and overall well-being.

Monitor Portion Sizes

Be mindful of portion sizes when reintroducing foods. Gradually increase serving sizes while staying attuned to your body's response.

Include Healthy Fats

Incorporate healthy fats, such as avocados, nuts, and olive oil, back into your diet. These fats are essential for overall health.

Reintroduce Dairy and Gluten Mindfully

If eliminating dairy or gluten, reintroduce them mindfully. Choose fermented dairy products and whole grains to assess tolerance.

Hydrate and Maintain Fiber Intake

Continue to prioritize hydration and maintain a diet rich in fiber to support digestive health.

Listen to Your Body

Trust your body's signals. If you notice adverse reactions or discomfort, reconsider the reintroduction of specific foods.

Maintaining Detox Benefits in Daily Life

Balanced Diet

Continue to prioritize a balanced and varied diet that includes a range of nutrients from different food groups.

Hydration

Maintain adequate hydration by drinking water, herbal teas, and other hydrating beverages throughout the day.

Mindful Eating

Practice mindful eating by savoring each bite, paying attention to hunger and fullness cues, and avoiding distractions during meals.

Regular Physical Activity

Incorporate regular physical activity into your routine to support overall health and well-being.

Stress Management

Continue stress-management practices, such as meditation, deep breathing, or yoga, to promote mental well-being.

Quality Sleep

Maintain a consistent sleep schedule to prioritize quality sleep.

Limit Processed Foods

Minimize the intake of processed and sugary foods in your daily diet. Opt for whole, nutrient-dense options instead.

Meal Planning

Plan meals ahead of time to ensure that they align with your health goals. This reduces the likelihood of making impulsive, less healthy choices.

Regular Detox Practices

Incorporate elements of your detox plan into your daily life, such as detox-friendly meals, herbal teas, and mindful practices.

Stay Connected to Your Body

Continue listening to your body's signals, adjusting your diet based on its needs, and staying attuned to your overall well-being.

Reflect and Adjust

Periodically reflect on your lifestyle, dietary choices, and overall well-being. Adjust your habits as needed to support long-term health goals.

Remember that sustaining the benefits of a detox is about adopting a holistic and balanced approach to your lifestyle. It involves creating habits that promote overall well-being, nourishing your body with wholesome foods, and maintaining practices that contribute to both physical and mental health.

CONCLUSION

Celebrating your detox achievement and embracing a lifelong wellness journey are significant milestones that deserve recognition and commitment. Here is a summary on how to celebrate your success and cultivate a sustainable approach to well-being based on everything we have discussed so far:

Celebrating Your Detox Achievement

Reflect on Achievements

Express Gratitude

Celebrate with a Healthy Meal

Pamper Yourself

Share Your Success

Create a Visual Reminder

Reward System

Capture Memories

Embracing a Lifelong Wellness Journey

Set Sustainable Goals

Mindful Eating Practices

Stay Active

Regular Detox Practices

Continuous Learning

Hydration Ritual

Regular Health Check-Ups

Community Engagement

Recognize that wellness is a journey, not a destination. Celebrate progress and be kind to yourself during moments of challenge.